DHEA

The Anti-Aging, Anti-Cancer and Anti-Obesity Hormone

Rita Elkins, M.H.

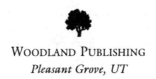

WOODLAND PUBLISHING
Pleasant Grove, UT

TABLE OF CONTENTS

INTRODUCTION

While scientists are slow to label any substance a "wonder drug," DHEA may very well be a therapeutic boon to the human body. Recent clinical tests conducted with DHEA have created a veritable flood of interest for both scientists and consumers. Estimates have placed the amount of in-depth clinical studies of DHEA at nearly 5000. These tests have been conducted at some of the most prestigious medical research centers and universities in the country. Unquestionably, DHEA is becoming known as one of the most important anti-aging and anti-disease substance of the 21st century among an impressive circle of scientists and medical professionals. Dr. Alan R. Gaby has stated:

> Current research suggests that DHEA may be of value in preventing and treating cardiovascular disease, high cholesterol, diabetes, obesity, cancer, Alzheimer's disease, other memory disturbances, and immune system disorders including AIDS, and chronic fatigue. DHEA may also enhance the body's immune response to viral and bacterial infections. . .New evidence suggests this hormone is so beneficial that it may turn out to be the most important medical advance of the decade.

DHEA: A Definition

DHEA is one of the most crucial and important hormones produced in the adrenal glands. It is frequently called "the mother hormone" because it constitutes the base for the biochemical actions of crucial hormones like testosterone, estrogen, progesterone and corticosterone. These key hormones along with others, control vital body functions which determine metabolism, energy output, endocrine mechanisms and reproductive capabilities.

In essence, DHEA orchestrates the entire endocrine system through a process of enzyme activation or inhibition. DHEA has very dramatically demonstrated an unusually wide spectrum of physiological benefits in many clinical studies. While scientists have known for years that the adrenal glands make DHEA, it has been only recently that its function in the body has been studied.

Sources of DHEA

The adrenal glands produce DHEA. It is also available as a non-patented prescription drug and in other over-the-counter forms. Many supplements include synthetic DHEA-S. Some consider Dioscorea extract found in Mexican Wild Yam as a natural source of DHEA. Naturally occurring compounds can mimic or precurse DHEA and do not presently require a prescription. Wild Yam or Mexican Yam can provide a botanical precursor of DHEA which is considered a valid source by some health advocates. Dr. Arthur Schwartz , an associate professor of microbiology at Temple's School of Medicine has conducted a number of studies using DHEA derived from Mexican Yam which is also called Dioscorea. Some controversy surrounds the clinical value of Wild Yam as a viable source of DHEA.

Action of DHEA

DHEA is utilized by the body to manufacture several other steroid hormones. It is the most dominant of all these hormones and contributes to the proper growth of brain cells, inhibits the conversion of carbohydrates to fats, decreases the formation of blood clots and helps to lower blood pressure. DHEA converts to or stimulates the production of estrogens, testosterone, progesterone, cortisone and other steroid hormones. Scientists have discovered that cells possess specific DHEA receptors which bind to DHEA, initiating a variety of biologic reactions.

Pharmacology

DHEA is short for *dehydroepiandrosterone,* which is a steroid hormone that plays a role in numerous biologic functions. It can:

>regulate hormones
>lower blood pressure
>decrease the stickiness of platelets that can clump and cause heart attacks and strokes
>increase estrogen in women and testosterone in men to youthful levels
>lower blood serum cholesterol (LDL)
>enhances overall immunity
>decreases the symptoms of an enlarged prostate
>helps to reduce menopausal symptoms
>promotes thermogenesis (fat burning)
>helps to increase muscle mass
>stabilizes blood sugar
>inhibits appetite and discourages eating
>boosts endurance
>inhibits diseases associated with aging
>can help restore collagen and skin integrity
>fights fatigue and depression
>helps to inhibit certain tumors
>improves calcium absorption which discourages osteoporosis
>acts as an anti-inflammatory

Therapeutic Applications

Research strongly suggests that DHEA can be used to prevent or treat a number of degenerative diseases including: breast cancer, high blood pressure, diabetes, obesity, and Alzheimer's disease. Recently its value for protecting HIV positive individuals from developing AIDS has emerged. It is also valuable for multiple sclerosis, chronic fatigue syndrome, memory loss, Parkinson's disease, high cholesterol, atherosclerosis, lupus, Epstein-Barr viral infections, osteoporosis, depression, menopause, herpes II, bacterial infections and as an overall anti-aging substance.

Normal Levels of DHEA

Males produce approximately 31 mg. Of DHEA every day and women, approximately 20 mg. Heredity is a significant determinator of how much DHEA we will produce. DHEA levels normally fluctuate within a 24-hour period by as much as 13 percent. In addition, DHEA levels seem to rise during the winter months

Causes of DHEA Depletion

DHEA levels can dramatically vary in each individual and can drop when the body is exposed to stress, or other conditions occur such as a plunge in blood sugar, fever, hypertension, nicotine ingestion, alcohol consumption and the presence of various diseases. In addition, taking birth control pills and other synthetic hormones can deplete DHEA levels. Drinking coffee can contribute to declining levels of DHEA in the human body. Consuming alcohol not only places more stress on the entire body, but decreases DHEA levels as well. Women who abuse alcohol have been known to have DHEA levels that were almost 40 percent less than non-drinking women. Even under the best of circumstances, the normal process of aging is a sure DHEA depletor.

Unfortunately, mental and physical stress along with these other factors can overtax the adrenal glands resulting in a depletion of DHEA. Some people have adrenals that are more resilient and resistant to common stressors, while others are extremely vulnerable.

When adrenal function is compromised all other endocrine functions are disabled including the production of DHEA.

NOTE: A vegetarian diet or the intake of saturated or unsaturated fats do not appear to significantly affect DHEA levels.

Substances That May Deplete DHEA

- coffee
- nicotine
- corticosteroid drugs
- beta blockers
- excess insulin
- alcohol
- synthetic hormones
- some hypertensive drugs
- calcium channel blockers

Substances Thought to Stimulate DHEA

- low blood sugar
- serotonin
- niacin
- tyrosine
- arginine
- lysine
- growth hormone
- GABA
- tryptophan
- phenylalanine
- ornithine
- melatonin

NOTE: People who routinely meditate and have learned to control and minimize stress have higher levels of DHEA.

Stress: Enemy of DHEA

The notion of high stress has been accepted as an inevitable and inescapable factor of modern life. While most of us are aware of how stress can raise cholesterol levels, initiate migraines, weaken immunity etc. the link between stressors and DHEA has remained relatively unknown. In addition, some clinicians believe that all disease is, in one way or anther, caused by the effects of stress. They believe that whatever region of body tissue is the most vulnerable or weak will most be adversely affected by stress.

Of particular interest is that any stressful event can depress the production of DHEA. These can include: surgery, physical trauma, strenuous exercise, death in the family, divorce, financial worries, public speaking, educational testing, re-location etc. Significant speculation exists among some health practitioners that DHEA levels may be disturbed in virtually every disease situation. While this may sound rather inclusive and unscientific, mounting evidence suggests that the role of DHEA in maintaining immunity is profound, to say the least.

In 1994, a Japanese clinical study intimated that "a disturbed balance between cortisol and DHEA-S could result in various aging and stress-related disorders."[1] Regarding another study with DHEA scientists recorded, "The present study provides direct evidence of the protective effects of DHEA as an 'anti-stress' agent."[2] DHEA is believed to actually protect the body against the brains reaction to stress. Studies have indicated that optimally, DHEA should be given prior to stressful situations.[3]

DHEA LEVELS AND DISEASE

Interestingly, low levels of DHEA have been linked to the development of various diseases including:

- arthritis
- cardiovascular disease
- atherosclerosis
- malignant tumors

- diabetes
- Parkinson's diseases
- chronic fatigue syndrome
- osteoporosis
- hypothyroidism

- Alzheimer's disease
- psychosomatic disorders
- disabled immune function
- chronic viral/bacterial infections
- hypoglycemia

Most of these diseases are invariable connected to aging as well; a fact that is more than just coincidental. If DHEA levels play such a profound role in health and aging, it only stands to reason that boosting declining DHEA levels could be very beneficial. If DHEA levels can signal the onset of certain age-related diseases and debilities, adding DHEA back to the aging body should counteract the biological effects of time to some degree. The next section of this booklet deals with specific diseases and how they may relate to and respond to DHEA therapy.

Diabetes

Anyone who suffers from diabetes also runs a higher risk of developing cardiovascular disease. Some studies have suggested that high levels of insulin cause DHEA to decline thereby
making diabetics susceptible to heart disease. Scientists are starting to believe that one reason why adult-onset diabetes and obesity occur in older individuals is due to their low DHEA levels.

Mice who developed diabetes and were given 0.4 percent dietary DHEA experienced a reversal of the disease due to the preservation of beta cells in the pancreas. DHEA has been able to lessen the severity of diabetes even when streptozotocin, a chemical which induces diabetes was administered to test animals.[4] Testing which was reported in 1995 using oral administration of DHEA found that it "enhanced tissue insulin sensitivity."[5]

These clinical studies have profound implications for anyone who may be susceptible to developing diabetes. The link between age, obesity and adult-onset diabetes may be intrinsically linked to declining DHEA levels.

Cardiovascular Disease

Elizabeth Barrett-Conner of the University of California states:

> A study of 242 men over the age of 50 found that those with high levels of DHEA in their blood were only half as likely to die of heart disease as those with relatively little of the hormone. Even with people without heart disease, DHEA seems to protect against early death. On its own, that's good news. But coming as it does after reports that taking DHEA can prevent or ease a variety of other illnesses, it may be the strongest evidence yet that a single hormone plays a contract role in maintaining human health.

Various other studies have confirmed the value of DHEA for the cardiovascular system. A study published in 1986 in the New England Journal of Medicine reported that men ages 50 to 79 were given DHEA supplementation which resulted in a 36 percent reduction in death from any cause and a 48 percent decrease in death from cardiovascular disease.

In 1993, a team of scientists tested DHEA's ability to inhibit coronary artery disease. They concluded, ". . .[DHEA] significantly retards the progression of accelerated atherosclerosis in both the transplanted heart and in the native heart."[6]

DHEA has been found to lower the level of blood serum triglycerides in several clinical studies.[7] The Department of Medicine at Johns Hopkins University reported in 1988 that increased levels of DHEA can stop the progression of atherosclerosis and reduce the risk of death from cardiovascular-related diseases. It specifically lowers LDL cholesterol which is the kind we don't want. Studies have shown that DHEA can accomplish this decline regardless of diet, exercise or weight modification. Again, the fact that low DHEA levels often accompany the development of heart disease must be considered. Apparently, DHEA levels initiate complex glandular reactions which ultimately determine the status or onset of many degenerative diseases.

Obesity

One of the most dramatic actions of DHEA has been seen in laboratory tests conducted on animals. The ability of DHEA to prevent the storage of lipids (fats) has emerged as another of its remarkable properties. The anti-obesity effect of DHEA has been significant, to say the least. Apparently DHEA helps to boost the changing of body fat to lean muscle, a process that becomes less effective as we age. DHEA can do what has traditionally been thought of as impossible; it can allow for weight loss without altering diet. In the presence of adequate DHEA levels, calories have more a tendency to convert to heat rather than to fat. DHEA seems to enhance the metabolic transformation of food into energy. This may explain why young people seem to readily burn calories, a process which seems to slow with age.

A research team which wanted to look at the potential of DHEA for treating cancer concluded in 1993 that, "Long term DHEA treatment of mice also reduces weight gain (apparently by enhancing thermogenesis) and appears to promote many of the beneficial effects of food restriction, which have been shown to inhibit the development of many age-associated diseases, including cancer."[8] The preliminary results of another study found that, "DHEA combined with a low energy, high fiber diet enhances the loss of excess body weight compared with diet modifications alone."[9]

In addition, how much DHEA we maintain may be involved in determining how fat is actually stored on the body.[10] Moreover, its relationship to insulin levels determined by blood sugar may help to determine hunger and fat storage. Recent evidence suggests that insulin levels may play a significant role in how much DHEA is actually metabolized.[11] Studies have discovered that low levels of DHEA may be related to an excess of insulin.[12] What this suggests is that anyone suffering from hypoglycemia or excess insulin, may be prone to converting nutrients to fat due to depressed DHEA levels.

Regarding weight control, additional studies found that DHEA did not cause any toxicity while it apparently stepped up metabolism and decreased both the number and size of fat cells.[13]

DHEA was given to five male, normal weight subjects at a dose of 1600 mg per day, divided into 4 doses. After 28 days, with diet and physical activity remaining normal, 4 of the 5 exhibited a mean body fat decrease of 31% with no overall weight change. This meant that their fat loss was balanced by a gain in muscle mass characteristic of youth. At the same time, their LDL levels fell by 7.5% to confer protection against cardiovascular disease.[14]

An Effective Appetite Suppressant

Not only does DHEA appear to step up thermogenesis (fat burning), it decreases the desire to eat. One study found that DHEA increased serotonin levels in the brain which resulted in less food craving.[15] Apparently our serotonin levels profoundly effect our moods, carbohydrate cravings, food intake and body fat. Several new studies have discovered that a desire to eat is not always based on true hunger. Frequently, neurochemistry determines when, what and why we want to eat. A persistent feeling of being hungry or not satisfied which can prompts incessant eating can be inhibited by serotonin synthesis and release within brain cells. DHEA stimulates the release of serotonin in the hypothalamus region of the brain, which reduces our desire to eat, thereby resulting in weight loss.

In 1995 a study was published which concluded that women who received DHEA as hormone replacement therapy decreased their food intake. DHEA was considered an appetite suppressant in that in significantly decreased the desire to eat.[16] Another recent study found that rats consumed a great deal more food after DHEA supplementation was stopped. "Upon removing dietary DHEA, rats immediately consumed significantly more food than while on the DHEA supplemented diets."[17] Another additional study concluded that "DHEA administration has an anti-obesity effect."[18]

Interestingly, the presence of fat itself may also contribute to the promotion of more fat by adversely effecting DHEA levels. One group of researchers concluded in 1991 that people with severe obesity are unable to increase their natural DHEA levels due to their high percentage of body fat. It is thought that this faulty mechanism contributes to the progressive accumulation of more fat and creates a vicious cycle.[19]

DHEA's involvement in thermogenesis or the burning of fat has been referred to as "energy wastage."[20] "Energy wastage is thought to be one of the ways that DHEA reduces body weight. . .Obesity and diabetes are characterized by high levels of gluconeogenesis, occurring in spite of increased levels of insulin . . . DHEA reduced gluconeogenesis."[21]

Unquestionably, the implications of DHEA therapy for obesity are profoundly significant and require further exploration. Initial test results strongly suggest the viability of using DHEA to help treat and prevent obesity.

Cancer

One of the most exciting therapeutic actions of DHEA is its potential for reducing the risk of developing breast, colon, lung, liver, and skin cancer. Dr. Schwartz originally became fascinated with DHEA when he learned that Dr. Richard Bulbrook had found that systemic levels of DHEA were consistently below normal in women who had developed breast cancer. Additional epidemiologic studies confirmed that the risk of developing a wide spectrum of cancers correlated to blood or urine levels of DHEA or DHEA sulfate.[22]

Other cancers that were associated with low DHEA levels were prostate, bladder and gastric cancer. Unlike the action of too much estrogen, DHEA has the ability to act as an anti-cancer agent. A clinical study published in 1995 in the *Journal of Cellular Biochemistry* found that by administering DHEA to laboratory mice and rats, tumors of the breast, lung, colon, liver skin and lymphatic regions were inhibited. Scientists conducting the study concluded that DHEA treatment not only inhibited the initiation of these tumors but kept them from developing as well.

They referred to the fact that substantial evidence exists the DHEA blocks certain biochemical pathways which generate oxygen free radicals which may initiate cellular mutations.[23] In other words, in these tests, DHEA inhibited the process necessary to initiate the growth of certain tumors. DHEA also inhibits an enzyme called G6OD, which can support the growth of malignant cells.

Additional testing with mammary tumors in mice found that DHEA may significantly reduce existing breast tumors.[24] Several of these tests have established a firm link between DHEA levels and breast cancer. Data indicating that DHEA was well below normal in a group of premenopausal women who had breast cancer substantiates this correlation.[25]

NOTE: Some tests found that under certain conditions, DHEA stimulated the growth of mammary and ovarian tumors or aggravated prostate disorders. This seeming paradox suggests that additional study of DHEA is more than warranted for the treatment of any tumor and that anyone suffering from hormonally-related cancers should check with their physician before taking DHEA supplements..

Autoimmune Diseases

Continuing research testing on DHEA has also discovered that the hormone may play a beneficial role in inhibiting the development of autoimmune diseases in which the body actually attacks itself. Several diseases fall into the autoimmune category and include: arthritis, Crohn's disease, some forms of colitis, and lupus. Much speculation exists that other diseases such as diabetes, multiple sclerosis, hypertension etc. may, in realty, be initiated by the autoimmune phenomenon.

Apparently, clinicians have found that serum levels of DHEA are frequently low in people suffering from rheumatoid arthritis and ulcerative colitis. Using DHEA therapy has resulted in significant improvement and suggests that DHEA for anyone with arthritis who also has a low DHEA level may be valuable. The use of DHEA for treating lupus has also recently emerged.

Lupus

A very recent open study of DHEA for the treatment of lupus obtained some encouraging results. Ten females who suffered from lupus were treated with oral DHEA for a period of three to six months. The research team concluded, "DHEA shows promise as a new therapeutic agent for the treatment of mile to moderate systemic lupus erythematosus."[26]

In addition, DHEA enhances the production of interleukin-2, a critical component of the immune system which is conspicuously low in people suffering from lupus. This particular correlation has prompted other studies using DHEA for multiple sclerosis as well. Initial data has been encouraging.[27]

AIDS

Multiple studies have shown the capability of DHEA to inhibit the reproduction of the HIV-1 virus. Evidently, DHEA has the ability to inhibit the replication processes of the virus while simultaneously boosting the immune response to viral invasion. In 1994, scientists discovered that DHEA could inhibit HIV-1 replication in vitro testing. They concluded that DHEA is " able to inhibit replication of both wild-type and AZT resistant HIV-1 . . ."[28] Concerning the use of DHEA as a viable treatment for AIDS, they stated [DHEA] may have a much broader spectrum of action than originally anticipated."[29]

Of interest is the fact that abnormally low blood levels of DHEA have also been associated with the stepped up progression of the HIV infection. In another recent study, 108 HIV-positive men with low T-cell counts were tested for DHEA levels. Those with blood serum levels below normal were 2.34 times more likely to develop AIDS that those whose counts were normal.[30] Clinical evidence of this kind strongly suggests that DHEA levels are depleted in people who are HIV positive, implying again, that DHEA plays a significant role in immune function.

Chronic Fatigue Disorder

Like AIDS, Chronic Fatigue Disorder is caused by a virus. The Epstein-Barr virus causes this particular disease, which is unusually difficult to treat. DHEA has been reported to protect against certain viral infections. It inhibits viral activity disabling its DNA synthesis in human cells. DHEA's ability to enhance the immune system is involved in this effect. Because of its association with boosted immune function, over the last few years, more and more physicians are looking to DHEA therapy for individuals suffering from Chronic

Fatigue Disorder. The ability of DHEA to boost energy and stamina has been documented.

DHEA: IMMUNE BOOSTER FOR DISEASE PREVENTION

Unlike other adrenocortical hormones, DHEA does not suppress the immune system. On the contrary, it is believed to stimulate T-cell production which potentiates the body's defense mechanisms. When we experience physiological stress, an excess of cortisol can result causing T-cell levels to drop. This explains the connection between physical trauma, surgery etc. and subsequent infections. The immune system becomes incapacitated to some extent, when the body is stressed. Boosting DHEA levels can help to counteract this effect.

Various research teams who have studied the many physiological effects of DHEA have found that it plays a significant role in regulating the body's immune responses.[31] DHEA has been tested on herpes, encephalitis and other infectious agents. Findings derived from these experiments strongly suggested that DHEA can help to protect against potentially fatal infections.[32]

A study published in 1995 strongly suggests that DHEA has the ability to reverse a weakened immune system and even protect the body from the influenza virus. By using DHEA vaccinations on aged mice, a significant increase in immune response was noted. In addition, enhanced resistance to direct exposure to live influenza virus was observed. The study concluded that DHEA treatment "overcame the age-related defect in the immunity of old mice against influenza."[33]

Scientists have concluded that DHEA can modify host resistance mechanisms rather than actually affect the virus itself. What this implies is that DHEA potentiates the body to more efficiently deal with physiological stressors and infectious invaders. Of particular interest is that anyone who has a poor immune response including older individuals, may specifically benefit from DHEA supplementation. Frequently, these people do not make adequate amounts of antibodies even when vaccinated. DHEA administered at the same time as the vaccination may help to boost antibody production.

DHEA Protects the Thymus Gland

It is the thymus gland which has the job of regulating the all-important T-cells of the immune system. Normally, immune mechanisms decline with advancing age during which the thymus gland simultaneously shrinks and becomes less active, resulting in more disease vulnerability. DHEA acts to protect and enhance the thymus gland by slowing down its degeneration. Controlled studies have found that DHEA has the ability to retard thymus gland atrophy under certain conditions. Some clinicians have even suggested that DHEA can actually stimulate the regeneration of thymus gland tissue, a claim that has not been scientifically validated as of yet.

At Last, A Fountain of Youth?

Since the beginning of time, the dream of sustained youth and prolonged life has been pursued by each generation. Today, scientists are just beginning to understand the physiological mechanisms which set our biological clocks. In the process, hormonal replacement therapies have emerged as the single most promising tool against aging. This type of protocol involves a complex therapeutic discipline which is still in the experimental stage. Its value, however, for the here and now should not be dismissed. The notion that we can prolong youth and prevent age-related disease is no longer considered an impossibility.

What has emerged as somewhat dubious is that if we eat right, exercise and learn to relax, we can postpone aging, remain lean and avoid a whole host of degenerative diseases. While this notion is a valid one to some degree, supplementing the body with a substance like DHEA has such a dramatic effect on human physiology that other practices pale in comparison. Research conducted over the last two decades has discovered that one of the most profound factors in determining how and when we age is our DHEA level. Many scientists even believe that DHEA has the ability to reverse aging to some extent restoring vigor and stamina, turning the clock back as far as is humanly possible at this stage in the game.

DHEA has the potential of working physiological miracles in terms of age-related disorders. One doctor at the Medical College of Virginia stated, "DHEA has become one of the most exciting developments in all of aging research."[34] Unfortunately, as time passes, the adrenal glands produces less and less DHEA due to the decreased function of an essential enzyme. By the age of 80, the adrenals manufacture only 5 percent of the DHEA they synthesized at age 20. More and more research indicates that a person's DHEA levels can be a predictor of his or her future health and longevity.

Dr. Samuel S.C. Yen of the UCSD School of Medicine has stated, "DHEA replacement in well-controlled human trials suggest that DHEA replacement has both psychological and physiological benefits for the aging population." Dr. William Regelson, an Oncologist at the Medical College of Virginia says, "As DHEA declines with age, you are losing the buffer against stress-related hormones. It is the buffer action of DHEA that helps prevent us from aging."

Dr. William Regelson, a medical oncologist at the Medical College of Virginia takes a daily dose of DHEA and has studied the hormone for 15 years. At 70, he looks and acts more like a man 20 years younger. As a strong advocate of DHEA replacement therapy, Regelson believes that DHEA can delay the physiological consequences of aging. Consider what Dr. Julian Whitaker, M.D. has to say about DHEA and aging:

DHEA is the mother load for some 18 different steroidal hormones integral to eternal youth. Unlike hormones that excite cells into activity, DHEA 'de-excites' the body's processes. Some of the diseases of aging are caused by the runaway production of nucleic acids, fats and hormones. DHEA slows down their production and thereby slows down aging.

Does Eating Accelerate Aging?

Interestingly, overeating has been singled out as one of the most significant contributors to a shortened life span. In the section discussing obesity, experiments with "undernutrition" found that by eating less calories and more nutrients, life could be prolonged. Realistically, most of us are not going to give up eating, however, DHEA may be able to accomplish similar results without forgoing food consumption. Dr. Schwartz has said that DHEA appears to be able to increase the transformation of food into energy, a process called thermogenesis.

Dr. Edward Masaro of the University of Texas Health Sciences Center in San Antonio recently stated, "If we can manipulate aging in the rat by nutrition, we probably can do it in any animal."[35]

DHEA AND LIFE EXTENSION

It is the regenerative capabilities of DHEA which have associated it with age reversal. Dr. Albert Schwartz, a professor at Temple's School of Medicine has conducted several tests with DHEA and has found that it was able to significantly prolong the life of laboratory mice. "When mice were fed DHEA, their life expectancy increased form 24 to 36 months; that is the equivalent of adding 35 to 40 years to the life of the average human. And the hormone appeared to add "quality" to those extra years. Mice fed the substance seemed younger and had a lower incidence of many of the traditional diseases of aging."[36]

Age-Related Physiological Changes

The process of aging inevitable results in declining levels of DHEA. Ample clinical evidence exists that replacing DHEA in men and women who were advancing in age exerted several significant benefits. The following conclusion was made after one study, "These observations together with the improvement of physical and psychological well-being in both genders and the absence of side-effects constitute the first demonstration of novel effects of DHEA replacement in age-advanced men and women."[37]

Menopause and DHEA

Because a drop in DHEA levels correlates with menopause, any symptoms associated with menopause may have a link to DHEA. One study showed that the average level of DHEA in premenopausal women was 542 as compared with 197 in postmenopausal women of which only 126 had undergone surgical removal of their ovaries.[38] These findings suggest that DHEA levels fall regardless of the hysterectomy factor, implying that the cessation of menstruation combined with other age-related changes diminishes endocrine output.

NOTE: Using natural progesterone cream has been found to actually raise DHEA levels.

Post-Menopausal DHEA Levels and Asthma

Very recently, a clinical study revealed that post-menopausal women who suffered from asthma had lower serum levels of adrenal steroids than other women their age who were not asthmatic.[39]

Osteoporosis

Because DHEA converts to forms of estrogen and testosterone when the body lacks these hormones, it has been singled out as beneficial for the prevention and treatment of bone thinning or osteoporosis. Some evidence exists which suggests that a decline in DHEA levels may well be correlated to bone loss that results from the aging process. Both estrogen and testosterone have shown beneficial effects for osteoporosis.[40]

In addition, progesterone also plays a significant role in the development of osteoporosis. One study did show that in a group of women between the ages of 55 and 85, a significant link between blood DHEA levels and bone density of spinal vertebrae was found.[41]

Because DHEA plays such an integral role in the synthesis of all of these hormones, it would not be surprising to learn that DHEA may determine the rate of bone loss which accompanies a decrease in other key hormones. Bone mass and fracture incidence studies have only recently commenced since the status of DHEA rapidly escalated from "mystery" hormone to "mother" hormone. These studies tell us that it is not aging alone which brings about osteoporosis. Current tests are even now strongly suggesting that supplementing DHEA to post-menopausal women may prevent the bone loss that accompanies osteoporosis.

DHEA and Calcium Absorption

The rate at which calcium uptake from the blood into the bones occurs may also be affected by the presence of DHEA. This would help to explain the role of DHEA in diseases like osteoporosis and arthritis. Hungarian experiments found that women suffering from osteoporosis had more trouble with calcium absorption. After receiving DHEA therapy, calcium which had stayed in the bloodstream was properly assimilated and metabolized. This study implies that just taking calcium supplements may not help to prevent or treat osteoporosis if DHEA levels are abnormally low.

Rheumatoid Arthritis and DHEA

Like, osteoporosis, DHEA levels have also been found to be lower than normal in women with rheumatoid arthritis.[42] Of interest is that taking cortisone drugs for arthritis pain decreases DHEA levels even more.[43] Combining test results with testing of DHEA links to osteoporosis once again supported the notion that blood levels of DHEA were able to predict bone mineral density. A fact which suggests a strong possibility that DHEA therapy may hold much promise for the treatment of rheumatoid arthritis. For anyone who has to take corticosteroids for arthritis, DHEA supplementation may also be of great value. Taking steroids appears to accelerate osteoporosis.

Increasing evidence is continually surfacing which also suggests that DHEA may directly impact the progression of arthritic disease. Some health practitioners have found it to contribute to a decrease in pain, inflammation and stiffness while boosting strength.

Dementia, Alzheimer's Disease and Cognitive Function

Dr. C.R. Merrill of the Laboratory of Biochemical Genetics in Bethesda, Maryland found that individuals suffering from Alzheimer's disease had 48 percent less DHEA than their healthy peers. In *Smart Drugs and Nutrients*, Dr. Ward Dean states, "DHEA protects brain cells from Alzheimer's disease and other senility-associated degenerative conditions."

Recent evidence published in the *American Journal of Physiology* found that DHEA may be valuable as a therapeutic treatment for age-related dementia.[44] Its effect on memory storage is related to how it modifies REM sleep. In addition, other studies have found that DHEA enhances memory retention and may improve cognitive function.[45]

A Sense of Well-Being

An article in the June, 1994 issue of the *Journal of Clinical Endocrinological Metabolism* stated:

> Patients and doctors are reporting that using DHEA as a dietary supplement promotes a youthful feeling of well-being and a much more positive outlook on life. In a 1990 study at the University of California Medical School at La Jolla, a group of men and women age 40 to 70 were given 50 mg. Of DHEA per day for six months. At the end of the study, 84% of the women and 67% of the men reported a remarkable increase in physical and mental well-being, energy, sleep, relaxation and ability to handle stress.

A study of forty-five post-menopausal women who had been on corticosteroids found that administering 20 mg. Of DHEA a day resulted in an increased sense of well-being with no side-effects.[46]

DHEA REPLACEMENT THERAPY

For many of us, the thought of hormonal therapy conjures up all kinds of concerns. For decades, the notion of taking hormonal elixirs has elicited all kinds of negative associations. While hormones are powerful molecules and should never be taken casually, little known hormones are emerging as the medicinal panaceas of the future. No one can ignore the scores of clinical tests which suggest replacing DHEA for its extraordinary physiological benefits. How long we live and our quality of life may be determined by supplementation with hormones like DHEA. Many advocates of DHEA are respected physicians and scientists who have recognized the enormous potential of this type of hormonal replacement and in many cases, have used themselves as test case studies. As is the case with any supplement, however, checking with your health care practitioner is strongly recommended before any therapy is initiated.

How Much is Enough?

Normal levels of DHEA are somewhere between 160 and 700 ug/dL. In an older person, 160 would be the expected reading, whereas for a 20 year old a reading of 700 is common. The ideal level of DHEA is thought to be between 500 to 700. Many clinicians believe if one's level is below 500, DHEA supplementation should be tried. If a woman's DHEA level is less that 180 ug/dL and a man's less than 220 ug/dL, or if any of the diseases discussed in the booklet are present, DHEA supplementation is highly recommended. A DHEA restoration protocol can be initiated under the supervision of a health care professional. DHEA doses depend on individual age and health and can dramatically vary.

Common dosages of DHEA used range from 3 to 35 mg. Per day. Initially, smaller doses are recommended with increases as needed. A high dose is considered over 25 mg. per day and should only be taken under the supervision of a health care professional, although doses of 50 to 100 mg. are not uncommon. Therapeutic doses of 1500 to 4000 mg. are used in cases of AIDS, multiple sclerosis or other serious illness.

Most practitioners recommend taking DHEA in several small doses throughout the day and alternating one day on and one day off.

For aging men and women, taking 100 mg, per day has yielded some remarkable results. Laboratory tests can measure blood levels of DHEA and DHEA-S, however, DHEA is not water soluble so its tissue level can fluctuate.

METHODS: DHEA can be taken in capsule form, placed directly under the tongue or taken in a liquid preparation which may be preferable for anyone with digestive disorders. Some home testing devices are available which can determine DHEA levels from saliva samples before supplementation is initiated.

SAFETY OF DHEA: DHEA appears to be remarkably safe even in relatively high doses, however, it is still considered an experimental drug and possible side-effects from its long-term usage have not been determined. Doses above 25 mg. per day should be monitored. While much evidence exists supporting the use of DHEA for cancer prevention, anyone with a pre-cancerous condition or any form of reproductive system malignancy should not use DHEA unless advised to do so under the careful monitoring of a professional health care provider.

NOTE: Some studies have suggested supplementing DHEA with vitamin E to help protect against any oxidation or liver stress.[47]

CONTRAINDICATIONS: Because DHEA is still considered an experimental drug, caution should be exercised. Anyone with ovarian, prostate or breast cancer should avoid usage. Possible side effects of DHEA include acne, increased hair growth on arms and legs.

CONCLUSION

At this writing, long-term, wide-scale testing programs with DHEA are currently in progress. The notion that DHEA supplementation may be one of the most profoundly beneficial therapies discovered to date is more than substantiated. Unfortunately, only a handful of physicians are aware of the benefits of DHEA. Currently, DHEA remains unpatented.

Consider Dr. Richard Passwater's prediction for the future role of DHEA: "Anybody over the age of 25 should be supplementing their diet with DHEA. One day this message will be endorsed by all medical experts. That is how important DHEA is to longevity."

ENDNOTES

1 M. Namiki, "Aged people and stress," NIPPON-RONEN-IGAKKAI-ZASSHI, February, 1994: 31 (2) 85-95.

2 Ben Nathan et al., "Dehydroepiandrosterone protects mice inoculated with West Nile virus and exposed to cold stress," J. MED-VIROL. November, 1992: 38 (3), 159-66.

3 C.N. Falany and K.A. Comer, "Human DHEA sulfo transferase: purification molecular cloning and characterization," DEHYDROEPIANDROSTERONE (DHEA) AND AGING, Meeting of the New York Academy of Sciences, June 17-19, 1995.

4 M.A. Jacobson, et al., "Decreased serum Dehydroepiandrosterone is associated with an increased progression of human immunodeficiency virus infection in men with CD4 cell counts of 200-499," JOURNAL OF INFECTIOUS DISEASES, 164, 864-68.

5 R, Casson, et al., "Replacement of Dehydroepiandrosterone enhances T-lymphocyte insulin binding in postmenopausal women," FERTIL-STERIL, May 1995: 63 (5), 1027-31.

6 D.M. Eich, et al., "Inhibition of accelerated coronary atherosclerosis with Dehydroepiandrosterone in the heterotopic rabbit model of cardiac transplantation," CIRCULATION, January, 1993: 87 (1), 261-69.

7 Casson, 127-31.

8 A.G. Schwartz and L.L. Pashko, "Cancer chemoprevention with the adrenocortical steroid Dehydroepiandrosterone and structural analogs," JOURNAL-CELL-BIOCHEM-SUPPL, 1993: 17 G, 73-79.

9 E.G. Macewen and I.D. Kurzman, "Obesity in the dog: the role of the adrenal steroid Dehydroepiandrosterone," J-NUTRITION, November, 1991: 121 (11 suppl), S51-55.

10 S.M. Haffner, et al., "Obesity, body fat distribution and sex hormones in men," INT-JOUR-OBESITY-RELATED-METAB-DISORDERS, November, 1993: 17(11), 643-49.

11 L Herranz, et al., "Dehydroepiandrosterone sulphate, body fat distribution and insulin in obese men," INT-JOURNAL-OBES-RELATED-METAB-DISORDERS, January, 1995: 19 (1), 57-60.

12 Ibid.

13 M. Cleary, et al., "Effect of dehydroepiandrosterone on growth in lean and obese Zucker rats," JOURNAL-NUTRI, 1984: 114, 1242-51.

14 "DHEA Replacement Therapy," LIFE EXTENSION REPORT, September, 1993, vol. 13, (9).

15 Ibid. 66.

16 C. Branco-Castelo et al., "Circulating hormone levels in menopausal women receiving different hormone replacement therapy regiments: A comparison," JOURNAL-REPRO-MED, August, 1995, 40 (8), 556-60.

17 J.R. Porter, et al., "The effects of discontinuing dehydroepiandrosterone supplementation on Zucker rat food intake and hypothalamic neurotransmitter," INT-JOUR-OBES-RELATE-METAB-DISORDERS, July, 1995: 19 (7), 480-88.

18 R. Sciborski, "The influence of DHEA on serum lipids, insulin and sex hormone levels in rabbits with induced hypercholesterolemia," GYNECOL-ENDOCRINOL, March, 1995: 9 (1), 23-28.

19 G. DePergola et al., "Low dehydroepiandrosterone circulating levels in premenopausal obese women with very high body mass index," METABOLISM, February, 1991: 40 (2), 187-90.

20 "DHEA Replacement Therapy," LIFE EXTENSION REPORT, 66.

21 Ibid.

22 Ibid., 67.

23 A.G. Schwartz and L.L Pashko, "Cancer Prevention with dehydroepiandrosterone and non-androgenic structural analogs," JOURNAL-CELL-BIOCHEM-SUPPL, 1995: 22, 210-17.

24 T.A. Ratco, et al., "Inhibition of rat mammary gland chemical carcinogenesis by dietary dehydroepiandrosterone or a fluorinated analog of dehydroepiandrosterone," CANCER-RES, January, 1991: 51 (2), 481-86.

25 B. Zumoff et al., "Abnormal 24-hour mean plasma concentrations of dehydroisoandrosterone and dehydroisoandrosterone sulfate in women with primary operable breast cancer," CANCER-RESEAR, 41, 3360-63.

26 R.F. Van Vollenhaven et al., An open study of dehydroepiandrosterone in systemic lupus erythematosus," ARTHRITIS-RHEUM, September, 1994: 37 (9), 1305-10.

27 V.P. Calabrese et al., "Dehydroepiandrosterone in multiple sclerosis: positive effects on the fatigue syndrome in a non-randomized study," in THE BIOLOGICAL ROLE OF DEHYDROEPIANDROSTERONE, edited by M. Kalimi and W. Regelson, New York, 1990: 95-100.

28 J.Y. Yang et al., "Inhibition of 3 azido-3 deoxythymidine-resistant HIV-1 infection by dehydroepiandrosterone in vitro," BIOCHEM-BIOPHYS-RES-COMM, June, 1994: 201 (3), 1424-32.

29 Ibid.

30 Jacobson et al., 864-68.

31 R. Morfin and G. Courchay, "Pregnenolone and dehydroepiandrosterone as precursors of native 7-hydroxylated metabolites which increase the immune response in

mice," JOU-STEROID-BIOCHEM-MOL-BIOL, July, 1994: 50 (1-2), 91-100.

32 R.M. Loria and D.A. Padgett, "Androstenediol regulates systemic resistance against lethal infections in mice," ARCH-VIROL, 1992: 127 (1-4), 103-115.

33 H.D. Danenbery, et al., "Dehydroepiandrosterone (DHEA) treatment reverses the impaired immune response of old mice to influenza vaccination and protects from influenza," VACCINE, 1995: 13 (15), 1445-48.

34 "Nutritional Information on DHEA," HEALTH STORE NEWS, Rolling Press, ref. File no. NSE-463-532.

35 Ibid.

36 Ibid.

37 A. Morales, et al., "Effects of replacement dose of dehydroepiandrosterone in men and women of advancing age," JOUR-CLIN-ENDOCRIN-METAB, June, 1994: 78 (6), 1360-67.

38 S.E. Monroe and K.M. Menon, "Changes in reproductive hormone secretion during the climacteric and postmenopausal periods," CLINIC-OBSTETRIC-GYNECOL, 20, 113-122,

39 R.E. Weinstein, et al., "Decreased adrenal sex steroid levels in the absence of glucocorticoid suppression in postmenopausal asthmatic women," JOUR-ALLERGY-CLIN-IMMUNOL, January, 1996, 97 (1 pt 1), 108.

40 "Hormone Therapy: Try estrogen/androgen in selected women," MODERN-MED, August, 1992: 60, 21.

41 R.A. Wild et al., "Declining adrenal androgens: an association with bone loss in aging women,"PROC-SOC-EXP-BIOL-MED, 1987: 186, 355-360.

42 P.N. Sambrook et al., "Sex hormone status and osteoporosis in postmenopausal women with rheumatoid arthritis," ARTHRITIS-RHEUM, 1988: 31, 973-78.

43 Ibid.

44 E. Friess, et al., "DHEA administration increases rapid eye movement sleep and EEG power in the sigma frequency range," AM-JOUR-PHYSIOL, January, 1995: 268 (1 pt. 1), E107-113.

45 J.F. Flood, et al., "Memory enhancing effects in male mice of pregnenolone and steroids metabolically derived from it," PROC-NATL-ACAD-SCI, March 1, 1992: 89 (5), 1567-71.

46 R.G. Crilly et al., "Metabolic effects of corticosteroid therapy in post-menopausal women," JOUR-STEROID-BIOCHEM, 1979: 11, 429-33.

47 M. K. Mcintosh et al., " Vitamin E alters hepatic antioxidant enzymes in rats treated with dehydroepiandrosterone (DHEA)," JOUR-NUTRI, February, 1993: 123 (2), 216-24.